The Secrets Of Going Natural

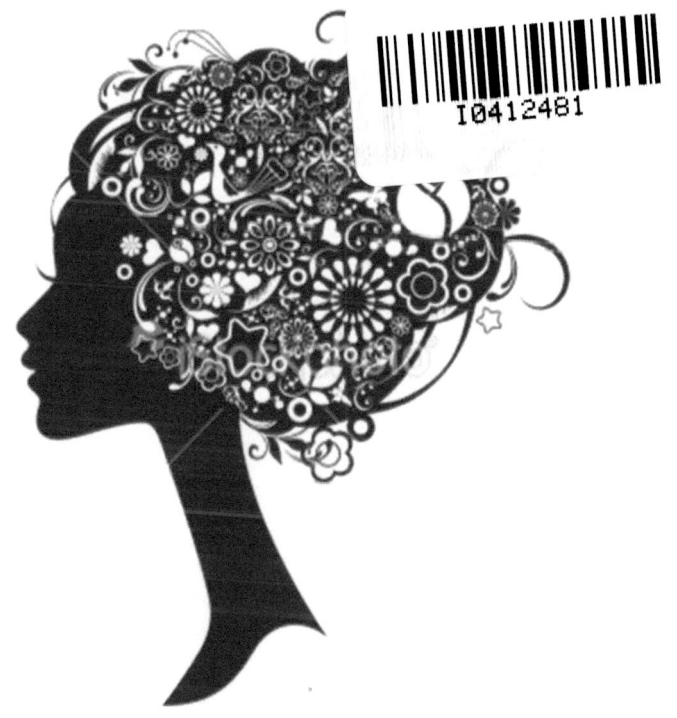

Zenobia Jackson

www.secretsofgoingnatural.com

DEDICATION

Dedicated to my awesome husband for inspiring me to write this book and for loving and accepting me for who I am. You'll never know how much you mean to me. I am so blessed to have you as my head, my husband, and my friend. I love You!

CONTENTS

ACKNOWLEDGMENTS

I would like to thank God Almighty for keeping His promises to me. He is not a man that He should lie. He continuously helps me to be patient with myself and others. Thanks to Sis. Joanna Holmes for her contagious "you can do it girl" spirit. Ms. Marissa Swan for exemplifying true sisterhood and for all of your honest thoughts, inputs, and work you put into helping make this book a success. To every woman I have talked to in the grocery store, shopping mall, gas station, gym and in the workplace, thank you for your stories of victories and defeats.

INTRODUCTION
Why This Book

After three years of being natural I can finally say, I am happy with my hair ☺!

Yes, it has been daunting at times but I have made it over the initial humps.

The problem I see now is that so many women I have come in contact with have not. And that makes me sad ☹.

I hate to see my beautiful sisters intimidated by the stereotypes of this world. Too afraid to take the leap and regain their naturally healthy hair.

So now, I am on the battle-field. Not for me this time, but for every woman out there who is warring with this decision of going natural. I intend to encourage and strengthen you in the trenches of this battle.

I want every woman contemplating going natural to know that they have a battle-buddy in the fox-hole with them. (Sorry, my husband was in the military ☺.

So step into my world of naturally healthy and beautiful hair.

Love,
Queen Z

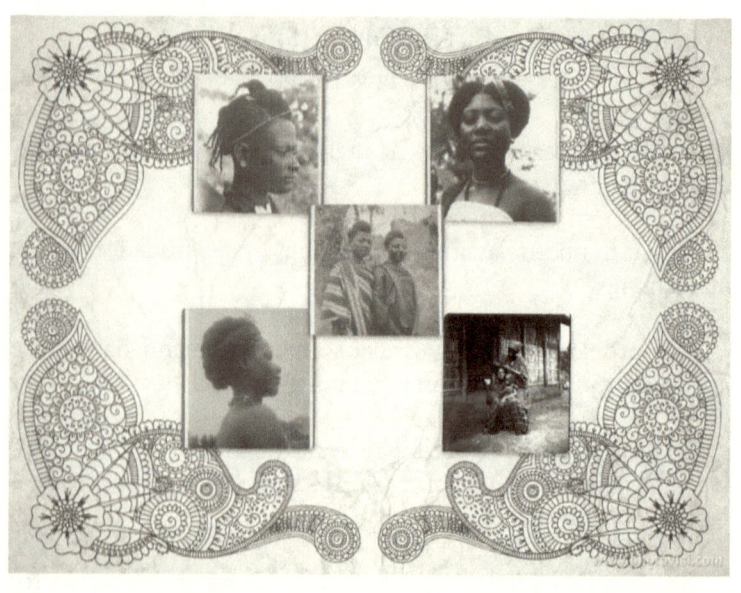

CHAPTER 1 ~ HISTORY OF NATURAL HAIR
Where It All Began

Nappy hair is a term people use for tangled or matted hair. This word can also be used when a person's hair becomes knotted and is very hard to brush out. In today's culture a woman with such hair is not looked upon favorably. In the beginning, our nappy hair was adorned and looked upon as a crown. It was a symbol of strength and beauty and not an unsightly mold.

Our hair was an outward expression of who we were as a people. Displaying every kink and twist brought a sense of knowing. Knowing who we were as naturally beautiful women.

In 1444, the Europeans discovered West African countries like Ghana, Liberia, Nigeria, and Senegal. These Europeans were not familiar with dark-skinned people nor were they familiar to the West African way of life. It is stated in the history books that in 1619 the first slaves were brought to Jamestown; an English settlement in Virginia. Our ancestors were 5,000 miles away from home.

They were in a strange and obscure place. Yes, it was strange for the Europeans, but I can imagine the thoughts and fears that raced through the hearts and minds of our people. How were they able to communicate with the Europeans? They did not communicate with them; instead they were kept silent and stripped of their identity. The

African language, culture and grooming traditions began to disappear.

Constant oppression of Africans slowly caused them to believe something was wrong with them. If you give this a little attention and place yourself during that time in history, you can imagine there was only so much oppression a man or woman could take.

In the 1800s, light-skinned, straight-haired slaves commanded higher prices at auctions than darker, more kinky-haired slaves. Internalizing color consciousness, blacks promoted the idea that blacks with dark skin and kinky hair were less attractive and worth less than those that were lighter.

We were not born hating the way we looked; rather we originally embraced our natural beauty for what it was. Racial self-perceptions began to change over time and we began to devalue our own naturally beautiful hair because of the opinions of others.

Sadly, this continues to be echoed today and evokes a skewed belief that if it isn't straight and curly, then it must be the opposite of good, thus, "bad" :-(

You remember don't you? The light-skinned kids with the "good hair". Can someone please tell me what "good" hair is?

In 1865: Slavery ends, but whites looked upon black women who styled their hair like white women as "well-adjusted".

"Good" hair becomes a prerequisite for entering certain schools, churches, social groups and business networks. So the idea of beauty has been distorted for over 400 years.

Who said words did not hurt?

They were talked about, beaten, families destroyed and dehumanized. They were the blackest, ugliest, and nappy, woolly headed animals on the planet. Africans, our people, were not given the right to be called human, simply because the Europeans feared what they did not understand.

My point in this brief historical enlightenment is not to start a riot, but to bring a sense of awareness and correct the wrong that has been done to our thoughts about our own appearance. The time has come to uproot the spirits of HATRED and FEAR and replace them with seeds of LOVE and ASSURANCE.

Why do we FEAR our nappy natural hair?

Or do we really just fear what others might think or say about our natural hair?

Who told you your hair was nappy? Who told you your natural hair was ugly and unattractive? Who told you that you were uneducated and stupid for having nappy hair?

To reiterate, fear is taught. It is a learned behavior. If you have ever been around a seven or eight-month old baby, you already know that you must watch them at all times. They have no fear, no sense of danger. They will pick up anything and place it in their mouth or touch something not knowing if it is hot or cold.

I imagined in my mind how it was before the Europeans invaded our ancestors' home. Mothers, sisters, and daughters content with their appearance, using exotic oils and herbs to twist and braid their daughter's hair and no one belittling one another because they accepted themselves for who they were; hair and all.

They were told, "you are beautiful, your skin is so soft, and your hair is glorious."

So I ask what teaching have you been listening too? We celebrate Madame C.J. Walker for her chemical treatments, and don't get me wrong: I admire her for standing strong and believing in her vision of chemical hair care products.

I don't judge her or any other woman whose choice is to chemically alter their hair.

My aspiration is to motivate those who have the desire to transition their hair back to its natural state. The issue no longer comes from the outside.

Today it comes from within. Free yourself from the world's perspective of beauty and begin to live your life as the natural Queen you were meant to be.

If this is you, you must begin to renew your mind daily and embrace everything about your natural hair.

Reflections of Chapter 1

1. Hatred and Fear must be uprooted and replaced with _____ and _____.

2. Fear is _____. It is a learned behavior.

3. True/False: I was not born hating the way I look.

List one major Fear in choosing to go natural.

FEAR _____.

Now combat that Fear with something Positive.

Love _____.

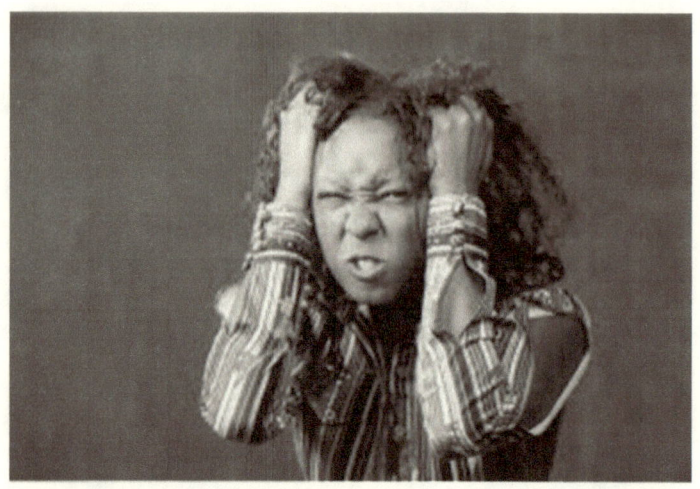

"My mind tells me to give up, but my heart won't let me."
~Anonymous

CHAPTER 2 ~ GET YOUR MIND RIGHT
Do You Have The Mental Toughness To Be Natural?

Is this really what I want to do? How will I look? What will others say? Will it be easy to maintain? Will it grow fast?

These are just a few of the questions that go through the minds of women who want to transition from permed hair to their natural hair.

Going natural should be based on your individual desire to have healthy, strong, virgin hair with the knowledge and expectation of a few bad "natural hair" days.

You must realize, as you make the transition, you are embarking upon gaining knowledge of your true self and true beauty.

Perming our hair over the years gave many of us a false sense of security. It was easy to brush it up into a ponytail or put a little heat in it to get some fire curls, but natural hair takes us into a different dimension. The way it feels and looks is so different than what we were used to, and now we must adjust our minds and hearts to love what we now see in the mirror.

To answer a few of your questions, such as, How will I look? You will look the way you've always looked! We must understand that as women we have a certain image in our mind of what we want to look like and when it doesn't look right to us, we will stop and do it all over until we think it is right. This is why some women go natural for one or two years then revert back to permed hair. We then say, "Girl... I tried that natural thing, but it just wasn't for me!"

I must say on a personal note there were many times I thought about going to Wal-Mart or the closest Target and buying a box perm, but a question always popped in my mind: Why? What is your reason for going back? Honestly, it was because of the way I felt about myself and what other women said to me.

My new look was not very welcomed in the beginning. So many people thought I had become depressed. They would say, "Your hair was so pretty, why did you do this to yourself". I laugh now, but then it was very hurtful. These insults came from those that I trusted and I valued their opinions.

I, like many other women, had that false sense of security. I no longer liked what I saw in the mirror and did not feel like I was attractive to my husband, not to mention all of the traditional women who thought I was crazy. If you ever decide to go back (and I pray you don't), let it be your choice and never the decision of someone else. Someone else's opinion of beauty should never become your truth.

Look into the mirror and ask yourself, "What is beauty?" My definition of beauty is a woman who has an inner strength that exudes from the inside out. The way she respects herself, that's beauty; takes care of her mind, body, and soul, that's beauty; sacrifices her time to benefit someone else, that's beauty; and bring other sisters up who may not be on her level, now that is simply beautiful.

So you see, beauty is deeper than what you or anyone else may see. Never allow anyone to dictate your change so that you can honestly say, "I tried it, but I just did not like it".

Choosing to go natural can expose many issues that we as black women thought we didn't have. Those issues can be insecurities, an unhealthy habit of pleasing others, and my least favorite, worshipping false idols, or idolizing other images. There is nothing wrong with valuing another woman's crown, but when you began to belittle the humble beginnings of your hair it becomes a problem.

If you admire a particular hair style or the texture of another sister's hair, compliment her and celebrate her achievements as well. It's all about loving yourself and others. As I stated earlier, it was easy to brush our hair up into a ponytail when we had a perm, but now we're trying to figure out what the heck we are going to do to our natural hair to make it look just as good as our old straight hair.

You may think you won't look the same and the question of how others perceive your hair will be there. What will my boss think? What will my friends and family say? You might feel as if your shell has been taken away from you, but in actuality your true beauty is being revealed. This is the hair God gave you. Whether it is soft and curly or kinky and coarse, it is your hair.

Instead of embracing our natural identity, we fight it and go through all kinds of unnecessary changes and emotional stresses.

When I talk about false idols, I'm speaking of the comments I often hear women make, such as "Why isn't my hair like her hair? Or "I wish I had her hair"!

Come on ladies; we must stop it! We are different, and beautiful in our own right. When the good Lord made you, He threw away the mold. There is no one like you, not even that beautiful crown that sits on your head is the same as anyone else's.

There may be similarities, but we have our own image, and now is the time to accept and embrace who we are. The hair is part of the package.

There is nothing wrong with admiring another sister's crown, but when we start purchasing everything she uses, thinking it will turn out exactly like her hair, we set ourselves up for disappointments. Not only are you disappointed, but now you are broke and mad at her. Our hair is just a piece of who we are, but it does not define us as women.

We should look at it as an art form just waiting to be expressed to the world. Genesis 1:26 says, "Let us make man in our image." Truth be told, our hair is important to

God, yet it is not everything. So why do we stress so much about the decision of going natural?

The 'image' reference that God was making was the totality of our person.

For me, the journey of going natural drew me closer to God because I had finally dealt with a personal fear of how others viewed me. Now I continue to thank Him for what He created. It was like an appreciation unto Him, which was long overdue.

God can use anything to bring Him Glory; and He used my hair! So ladies I want you to know you are beautiful. Whether you have short, kinky or long and wavy hair, you are beautiful. Make up your mind today and choose to be free inside and out!

Reflections of Chapter 2

1. Going natural should be based on your
   _____desire to have _____ &
   _____ virgin hair.

2. Choosing to go natural can _____ many issues
   we as black women thought we did not have.

3. True/False: There are many similarities and many
   differences in our hair because we have our own
   image.

   Define *BEAUTY* in your own words.

   _____

   _____

   _____

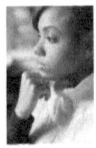 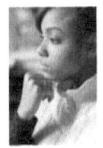

My Personal Thoughts

_____

_____

_____

_____

_____

_____

_____

_____

_____

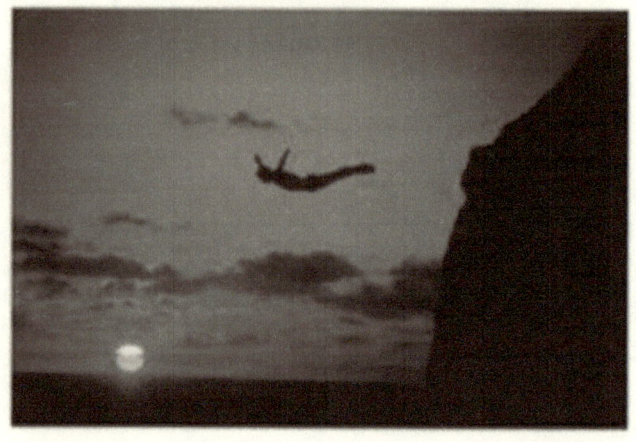

"Don't put off until tomorrow what can be done today."
~Anonymous

CHAPTER 3 ~ THE JUMP OFF
Choices, Choices, Choices

So you have decided to do it, huh?

Then here is where we talk about how to make it happen.

There are three main forms of transition that I want to discuss in this chapter.

The first is the BC also known as the "big chop". This is when you cut all permed hair completely off. You may decide to shave it or leave only the new growth, which is the virgin (natural) hair. The BC is recommended for those sisters who are wiping the slate clean.

Some women are bold and take the "leap of faith" by cutting it all off, not considering how others view them. These are the Radical Queens! Radical Queens know what they want and have a healthy conscience and image of who they are. Hair to these women is an art and they can't wait to show off the next Monet.

There is little work to be done using this type of transition, yet at this point you will begin to nurture your hair by finding out your hair type and keeping a clean scalp. Many women feel comfortable wearing a low-fade as their hair grows blossoming into a TWA (teeny-weeny-afro).

This is the beginning of having healthy, happy hair; and healthy, happy hair is strong, resilient, growing hair. We will talk later on hair type, but for now let's focus on the second type of transition.

The second and third transition or method of wearing your hair focuses on the growth of your natural hair. When using this type of transition many women go through a "transition period". Transition takes place when you make a mental decision to no longer use chemicals on your hair that changes its texture. This includes relaxers, texturizers, or curly perms.

You may decide not to cut all your permed hair off, and that is okay. The second method (**Braids**) will allow your new growth to continue to grow underneath the permed portion and start the journey to one day exposing your natural hair.

Many women have said their hair has grown faster by wearing braids. Transition methods include wearing braids, weaves (preferably sew-ins), wigs, or rodding your hair.

Don't worry ladies, you won't lose your natural sister points for this. It boils down to what is comfortable for you during this phase. This may be easier for some women, instead of just rocking a TWA (teeny-weeny-afro) as seen with many BC transitioners.

As long as you keep a clean scalp, i.e.: washing it regularly, applying a moisturizer and massaging your scalp (which increases blood flow), your hair will grow.

Famous hairstylist for the stars, Diane Da Costa and author of "Textured Tresses" says, "Hair relies on the bloodstream for its life and health; similar to plants, which depend on the nutrients absorbed by the soil" (Da Costa 17).

Yes, it may be time consuming, but anything worth having, takes sacrifice. You don't have to massage you hair every night, rather two to three times a week will be a great start. You may still be adjusting and embracing the new you and this is okay.

My personal process on becoming natural consisted of both transitions. I wore braids for an entire year. Braids gave me more flexibility for my lifestyle. I wore them in three-month phases. During those three months, I washed twice a month and applied Medicated Nextimage 5 in 1 Itching Free Conditioner. It was a spray that consisted of olive oil, jojoba oil, shea butter, and Tea-tree oil.

After that year, I did the BC and did not feel comfortable with the short length, so I wore braids for about three months and switched to sew-ins. My hair grew ridiculously long and thick. It had grown to the point where

I could create my own art. However, wearing braids can also cause hair and scalp damage, so be careful.

Many women do not realize that while length can be beautiful, having long, heavy extensions puts additional pressure on the scalp. This pressure can pull your hair out, and may cause long-term damage in the form of thinning and pre-mature balding.

Therefore, if you are trying to grow your hair long, you might want to think seriously of the potential hindrances hair extensions could pose to your long-hair quest.

Here are the 3 tips concerning braids:

- Tip # 1 Never get extensions that are down your back. The longer the braids, the more stress and pressure your scalp will be under- which will cause breakage.

- Tip # 2 Make sure your stylist does not braid your edges tight. Around this area is very sensitive. The hair around your temple is soft and fragile and easy to break.

- Tip # 3 Keep your scalp clean. Whether you wash your entire head or wipe with a soft astringent such as Witch Hazel, keep it clean! Also apply a moisturizer to your hair even while it is braided.

This is how I had great success in rocking my twists for an entire year and was able to achieve growth. So as I began to wear and style my natural hair, my creative visions began to flow. Whether it was an original masterpiece or an inspiration from a sister off of YouTube, I was and will forever be excited and loving my natural hair.

For those that immediately have fallen in love with their natural TWA and want the world to see: I congratulate you.

The third type of transition is wearing a weave. **Weaves** can be a great protective style if done properly. Wearing a weave allows your hair to "rest" as it grows. However, if you are considering adding a weave to your natural hair, it will be very important to explore your options and understand the different effects that certain hairstyles can have on your natural hair.

It is also imperative that you take precautions to minimize the risks of damaging your natural hair and scalp. You must know the difference between synthetic (plastic) hair and human hair in order to accomplish the desired look. The synthetic is best for braids while the human hair is more suitable for use of free-flowing styles.

There are many types of human hair to choose from: Asian, European, and Virgin/ Raw hair. Your personal preference, hair type, and cost restrictions will determine what type of extensions you and your stylist should choose.

Rodding your natural hair is simple. Some sisters completely stop perming their hair and began to rod it or do what we call "sister curls". Eventually, they cut the permed hair off and began to style the natural hair.

Even in this transition, conditioning the hair is important because there will be a lot of shedding. Your scalp will be freaking out because it will crave the chemicals that it was once accustomed to having every two to three months, and for some women, every month (yikes). Pay attention to Appendix D concerning the truth about perms.

Texturizers are another means of transitioning. Many women opt for chemical processes that loosen the curl with a softener or texturizer because it makes the hair a little easier for to them to manage and to add some curl definition to really curly, coily, or kinky hair.

What exactly is a *texturizer*? It is a mild relaxer. It is applied in a specific way so as to avoid removing the natural curl formation from the hair. Some have sodium hydroxide, also known as lye, which is also in drain cleaning agents for clearing clogged drains!

Using this type of texturizer will require that your scalp is based. Basing your hair is the application of petroleum/Vaseline to the scalp in order to protect the scalp from burning or becoming irritated. This practice is used before the perm is applied to the hair/scalp and to ease burning if one has previously scratched their scalp. Also, a no-lye relaxer can be used as a hair texturizer for kinky, curly, or coily hair.

This type of relaxer works well for those with a sensitive scalp. However, no-lye relaxers can also be somewhat drying to the hair, unlike lye relaxers. Your scalp must also be based for this type of relaxer.

There are pros in having texturized hair. It gives you control and manageability in styling your hair. It also reduces the frizziness that comes from natural hair that may be kinky or curly. The con is the very fact that a texturizer is a chemical. No matter how you slice it, texturizers change the natural state of your hair - and we don't want that ☺

You must remember the definition of natural hair as being symbolic to the term "virgin". Natural hair is pure and untouched. It should not be stripped from its natural state and texturizers to an extent change the natural state of the hair.

My personal opinion is that if a woman decides to use a texturizer, it is her choice, but I don't consider them natural at all. Natural to me is having unprocessed hair and using hair products if containing chemical additives will not damage the hair. Remember, this is my personal opinion.

So now you have the information you need to make an informed decision about the best way to make the transition for you.

Reflections of Chapter 3

1. There are three methods of transitioning.
   List them: _____, wearing _____,
   and/or wearing _____.

2. Natural hair is symbolic to the term _____.

3. True/False: A texturizer does not change the natural
   state of your hair.

   Which transition have you chose and why?

   _____

   _____

   _____

   _____

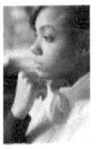 My Personal Thoughts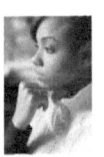

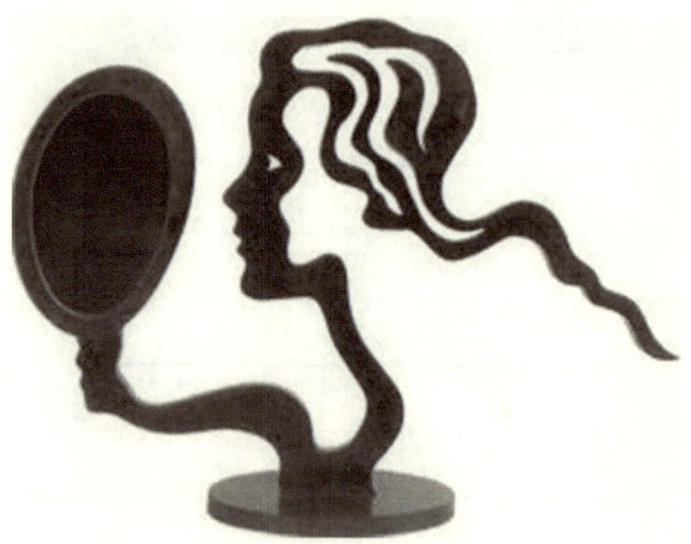

Mirror, Mirror, on the wall,
is this the type of hair I have after all?

CHAPTER 4 ~ I THOUGHT I HAD GOOD HAIR
What is 'good hair'?

Does this sound familiar? "*I thought I had good hair*"!

Many women have had a reality check since their "jump off" experience– their period of beginning the leap into natural hairdom. They see something that may be a tad different than what they envisioned for their natural hair to be, look, or even feel. That is because for many of us transitioning from permed hair, to having natural hair, we have never seen our hair in this state before. Natural hair has a unique look. A look of confidence and acceptance.

Let me ask the question, "*What is good hair?*" Well, let me first tell you what it is not. Good hair is not soft and curly, good hair does not wave up when you add water only. Good hair is not long and straight.

Again, we have this misconception of what "good hair" is. Whether it is what we have seen on television or what we have heard others say, or even our own vain imagination, good hair is simply healthy hair! You do not have to have soft nor curly hair and it certainly does not have to flow down your back.

Now before someone begins to think I am "hating" on sisters with soft or curly hair, I am not. I am simply erasing the images of what good hair is. I admire women who have all types of hair. Short, long, coarse, and fine. I especially love to see women who have embraced their specific hair type and rock it like only they can. Good hair is growing healthy hair; it is hair that you have taken the time to nurture in ways never imaginable.

So ladies, in order to achieve your good head of hair, you cannot be lazy, nor can we afford to be ignorant. Now don't get offended. *Ignorance* is simply the lack of knowledge or information. I've been there before and this is the whole purpose of this book: to help you avoid many of the mistakes I made.

The most vital part of going natural is knowing and understanding your hair type. Do you know your hair type? Most women do not. I was planning my interviews for this book and I asked a young lady who had short beautiful hair what her hair type was and she began to tell me the type of color she had in her hair. She really did not have a clue on what I was talking about. We must know that in every aspect of our life we will perish without knowledge and the application of it.

Something we may think is simple or really not important may be the very thing that leads us to failure. Not knowing your hair type will cause you to hate your hair instead of loving your hair. You will spend more money on your hair now than when you had a perm.

You will be forever in search of what works for you. That is one of the biggest issues many women face - spending unnecessary money on high-priced products because the products seemed to work so well for another sister. Da Costa says, "Your natural hair texture is going to be dramatically different, yet you have to be comfortable with yourself and believe that you look gorgeous no matter how your hair looks. You are not your hair." I could not agree more.

In Appendix A I have included a quiz to help you figure out your hair type and texture along with products that will aid in your healthy hair journey.

Reflections of Chapter 4

1. Good hair is _____ healthy hair.

2. The most vital part of becoming natural is
    _____ & _____ your hair type.

3. True/False: Ignorance is simply the lack of
    knowledge or information.

What was or is your perception of "good hair"?

_____

_____

_____

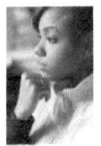 My Personal Thoughts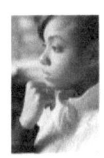

_____

_____

_____

_____

_____

_____

_____

_____

_____

_____

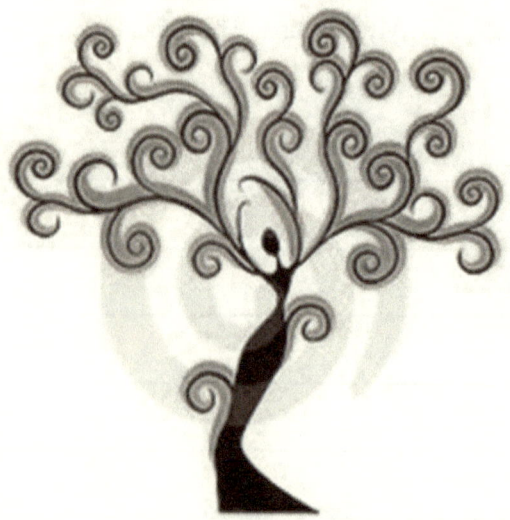

"In the middle of difficulty lies opportunity."
~Albert Einstein

CHAPTER 5 ~ THE 3 P'S OF NATURAL HAIR
Patience, Persistence, & Positivity

I have found that taking this journey into loving our God given hair can cause us to grow in many ways. Whether you are timid and doubtful or bold and sure, there are three bridges we all must cross in order to receive freedom.

The first bridge is called Patience. Patience is understanding your hair and caring for it. I had been praying to God to help me with patience with my family, co-workers, etc. Just recently He revealed to me how I can be patient. He said, "STOP and pay attention to what is going on.

I have three wonderful, smart, handsome boys and there are times when they all want my attention at once. All I can hear is, "Mama, mama, mama". My normal reaction is to scream, "BE QUIET" without stopping to see about them in a caring and loving manner.

My boys are my heart, but I know there have been times when they felt like I was the worst mom in the world, and that is because of my reaction to their needs. I should have entered their world in a graceful manner, calming them down and giving them what they needed, which was my undivided attention.

This is what we have to do concerning our mane. Realize that your hair has changed. You no longer have a perm, so your normal regime has to change. Pay attention to the changes in your hair. Read, research, and experiment with products, but accept your tresses for what they are. The reality is perm hair is different from natural hair and should be cared for accordingly.

On your head you may even have two different types of hair textures and your growth may vary. My hair is super coarse in the center of my head and not as long as the back. The back seems to grower faster, but I no longer become frustrated with my hair; I let it do what it's going to do.

I am patient with my hair. Every style is not for me, every product is not for me. This I learned through trial and error.

June 2011, I will have been natural for three years and it has not always been easy. Patience is mastered over time, and the time when you want to head to your local Wal-Mart or call your beautician for a perm that is when the choice will come, to be patient with your natural hair or give in to the pressures.

The second bridge is Persistence. Persistence is the continuation of something; not giving up. My husband is the epitome of this word as I watch him work tirelessly on those things that are of importance to him. He wakes up every morning at 5:30 to spend time with God in prayer and thanksgiving. Thinking about his students and how he can better himself in the classroom also spending more time with our boys every chance he gets. Now if that isn't persistence then what is?

We as a people rarely stick with anything that requires more skill or patience than we currently have. If it doesn't turn out the way we think it should turn out, we give up! To be honest, it is much easier to give up. This is the reason so many of us do give up. When it comes to your hair it's the same way. Your environment plays an important part of your persistent attitude.

I have always had a carefree attitude. I never went with the crowd, so to speak. I did things because I chose to, whether those choices were good or bad. I took to those choices and learned from every one of them. I can remember in pre-school, I would put my lipstick on, along with my plastic pink and purple heels in my little backpack. As soon as my mom would drop me off, I would go into the girl's restroom and change into a little diva.

The teacher would always ask me, "Does your mother know you're wearing lipstick?" I would smile and nod my head implying yes. As I grew older, my perception of a lot of things changed and I subconsciously began to care about the views of other people until I lost myself. The corruption of videos, magazines, and other women's opinion of beauty entered my mind and distorted it, but today I am free again.

My carefree attitude has changed from not caring about myself to caring about what's best for me and the ones I love. I have that freedom again of just being me the same way a child does! If you have decided to start your natural hair journey, you must be persistent. You may ask how?

First, realize that your hair is NOT you, but it's a part of you.

Accept this fact and embrace your God-given crown. It is up to you to take care of it just like every other part of your body. It doesn't matter what hair type you have - know and believe that you are beautiful! If you haven't realized it yet, let me be the first to tell you,

YOU ARE BEAUTIFUL!

I believe God wants you to nurture and care for every beautiful straight, kinky or curly strand on your head. When we as women begin to understand that neither things nor people make us, nor have we made ourselves, but that our Heavenly Father who is in heaven has made us and love us for who we are and what we look like, THEN we will be able to reign as Queens.

Secondly, do not allow the nay-sayers keep you from your hair destiny.

If I had a dollar for every person who told me how ugly I was going to look, that my hair was not going to grow, or asked that infamous question, "**When are you going to perm your hair**", as if my decision to go natural was a joke, I could take a nice little trip to the Bahamas. You must expect and welcome these offensive statements. Many of them come from an ignorant perspective on beauty.

People that make these statements simply don't know you and don't understand where you are going. They have a definition of what beauty is and often it is a skewed one.

Whether it's your husband, sister, brother, co-worker, or a complete stranger, you may choose to explain your reason for going natural in order to enlighten those who are curious. Some of you may not see the need to explain, but which ever you choose never be rude. I feel if you do choose to explain to others about your decision to go natural, just know that you may be helping others see beauty from a perspective they didn't have before. However, while some may understand, others may continue to fight against your decision.

You may be thinking, "It can't be this serious". It may not be as hard for you to transition, but many women face the crowd of nay-sayers.

There was a woman who came to visit me on my job and had been natural about a year. She loved the style I was wearing and wanted to know about my process. She loved her decision to go natural, but her husband was totally against it. She told me he had made an appointment for her to get a perm. She was heartbroken.

I can only imagine the thoughts going on in her mind. I am not an advocate of a wives being disrespectful and not honoring their husband, yet, it amazes me how something as simple as hair can cause friction within a marriage.

Saying all of this, I do believe in prayer, and a heartfelt prayer as simple as "Lord strengthen me as I go on this journey of loving me and help those around me to see me as **You** see me" can break the strongest man.

This prayer not only refers to a marriage, but any relationship you may have. I learned that our biggest concern comes from those who are closest to us - family and friends. So be strong and be persistent!

The third bridge is Positivity. Have you ever heard the saying, "You will only be the average of whom you surround yourself"?

This is true in every aspect of our lives. If you're constantly around people who are not supportive of you going natural, it is more likely that you'll resort back to your traditional way of hair styling. Resorting because of others is always bad if it's not for the betterment of you. After all, it's your hair.

When we fold to the pressures of other people's demands or thoughts of us, they are in control. Again, the matter of a marriage has a different antidote, but for everyone else, they don't have the right.

Now my belief concerning a marriage is that if your husband is totally against this journey on going natural, God has already given you the power of persuasion. The power of persuasion and manipulation are two different things. Our power of persuasion is used so that God may ultimately get the glory.

So ask yourself, why have I decided to go natural? In the beginning, my reason was because of the effects of having permed/colored treated hair. Over the years, it had become thin, weak, and dry. My prayer was "Lord should I do this?" and in asking Him, He asked me a very simple question, "Why?" Then and only then did the layers begin to peel off. It was so much deeper than hair.

My husband understood my reasons and supported me. So for those that are married, my answer to you is prayer. Proverbs 21:1 says, *"God has even the king's heart in His hand"* so I am sure your husband's heart is there also. Our home should be a positive place to share and embrace our differences. As for outsiders, allow them to have their opinions, but do not let their opinions have you.

In fact, God promises to strengthen you as a person when you encounter opposing opinions with courage – "Have I not commanded you? Be strong and courageous. Do not be afraid; do not be discouraged, for the LORD your God will be with you wherever you go" (Joshua 1:9). So consider it joy when you encounter any trial and be courageous!

There is a whole world filled with sisters taking the leap of faith, believing in spite of others, I am going to do me! I want you to realize something my Queens: there is no one like you. You were made by the hands of God himself. Your uniqueness deserves to be seen throughout this earth.

There is a network of natural sisters all over this world; from France to the Bronx. Women are going back to the basics and embracing their "nappiness". Submerge yourself around other natural sisters and learn from them. Ask questions and listen to their stories, and most importantly, encourage one another by staying positive. Positivity eventually erases negativity.

To be honest, some sisters may discourage you because they want to take the leap of faith themselves. You would be surprised at the number of reasons why going natural is not looked upon favorably.

Regardless of the reasons, I encourage you to show off and show out. Continue to be positive in every area of your life and see your expectations become a reality for you. See your hair growing, becoming healthy, and resilient.

Would you imagine all of these results (healthy, growing hair, and more importantly, personal strength) coming from crossing the bridges of patience, persistence, and positivity? I have and continue to cross these bridges every day with my hair. It has become normal for me, and anything done long enough becomes a habit.

Let us began to care for our hair in a habitual manner. Making time to stop and listen to the needs of your hair, continuing to press toward your goal in achieving healthy natural hair, and keeping a wonderful attitude even when you have a bad hair day. Grab hold toward your natural destination and never let go.

Reflections of Chapter 5

1. The three bridges in having natural hair are
_____, _____, & _____.

2. Positivity eventually erases _____.

3. True/False: Our gift of persuasion is used to manipulate others.

Think of a time when God carried you through a situation. How did you feel when you made it through?

_____

_____

_____

_____

Note: Our hair is NOT bigger than God.

CHAPTER 6 ~ THE TOP 10 QUESTIONS
Questions Transitioners Ask

Here is a list of questions women have asked when deciding to transition. Of course, not every question is here, but I chose the top 10 that I thought would get you off to a great start!

Question 1
Do I have to cut all of my permed hair off?

~Absolutely not. It is truly your preference. Some women do the "big chop", that is, cutting all permed hair off, while others wear extensions, weaves, or wigs. My opinion is to do whatever is comfortable for you. Doing what's most comfortable for you will greatly help your transition be easier, so that you don't feel as tempted to revert back to permed hair. I wore braids a year, then I cut the remaining permed hair off.

Question 2
Is it normal for my scalp to be itchy and sore during my transition?

~ Yes it is! Your scalp has been addicted to perm for as long as you had one, and now you're not feeding it. It is similar to an addict trying to go "cold turkey". They become irritated with themselves and others. My scalp got very, very sore for about two months. My hair was going through withdrawals. I kept my scalp clean and gave myself daily massages. Hang in there!

Question 3
Will I be able to comb through my natural hair?

~ Of course. Natural hair can be combed throughout its entirety, but make sure it's fully wet and saturated with a conditioner. Knowing your hair type also allows you to know how to comb your hair with minimal breakage. Women who have type 2 hair (Fine, thin and manageable) may find comb usage to be a breeze, but as hair types vary, so do styling methods.

I have 4a type hair (coarse tightly coiled hair) that, when stretched, has an "S" pattern). I finger comb my hair mostly. Finger combing is when you use only your fingers to section and comb through your hair. This is a great way to maximize your natural curl definition.

Question 4
What is a "no poo" ?

~ It stands for the "no shampoo method" of haircare, which means that when you wash your hair you don't use shampoo to wash, but use conditioner instead- sometimes enriched with baking soda or lemon. This method is popular with natural haired women, because traditional shampoos, especially those containing sulfates, will dry out afro-type hair very easily. I use neutralizing shampoos for ridding my hair of air pollutants and dirt. Clarifying shampoos are known to be harsh on natural hair. If you decide to shampoo, read the labels. Stay away from products that have alcohol in them. It will dry your hair.

Question 5
Should I still go to a salon to assure the overall health of my hair?

~ This depends on your expectation and the personality of your hair. Cutting, coloring, and certain styles should be cared for by an expert. I know for most of us, going natural was in order to stay away from the beauty salons, but we should seek the advice of others who have invested time in properly caring for natural hair. My hair regimen now is pretty simple. I go to the salon only twice a year to clip my ends, wash once a week, moisturize daily, twist before going to bed and rock it if I'm going out. As long as those ends are clipped, and your scalp is clean, your hair will retain its length.

Question 6
Do I have to press my hair to clip my ends?

~ No. Whenever I go to see my beautician she cold washes my hair, saturates it with conditioner and clips the ends. She is also natural and has 15 years of experience with natural hair. I trust her, but you can press your hair if you prefer. It is a personal decision and one I encourage you to do minimally. Too much heat can and will damage your hair and strip your hair of its normal curl pattern.

Question 7
What causes *fairy* knots and how do I get rid of them?

~ For those who may not know what fairy knots are, they are tiny knots at the ends of your natural hair; single strands close to the ends of natural hair. They are caused by the hair having a tight curl pattern which results in the hair wrapping around itself resulting in a tiny single-strand knot. You will never get rid of all fairy knots, but you can alleviate most of them. Here are five simple tips:

- Seal your ends every night with shea butter, coconut oil, olive oil, or jojoba oil.

- Do not comb dry natural hair. Only comb or finger through your hair when it is wet and saturated with conditioner .

- Wear protective styles often.

- Always tie your hair down at night with a satin scarf to prevent matting, tangles, abrasion of hair strands against rough surfaces, and drying of the hair from absorption by cotton pillowcases.

- Condition often – every time you wash, meaning at least once a week.

Question 8
I have dry hair. What can I do?

~Condition, condition, condition! You hair needs to be hydrated daily. Just like our bodies need water, our hair needs conditioning. Two of my favorite conditioners are: "Shea Almond Coconut Deep Cream Conditioner" and "Desert Moisturizer & Leave-In Conditioner" by Bear Fruit Hair. Great products, great price. You can also see Appendix B for my other product recommendations.

Question 9
Is it okay to color my hair, and if so, what works best on natural hair?

~Personally, I believe it is completely safe to color your natural tresses. There are three brands that have gotten rave reviews from other women who have natural hair. EcoColors, Herbatint, and a semi-permanent natural hair color by Herbatint called Vegetal. Check them out and see what works for you. When coloring your hair, I recommend a professional (a colorist) to add the color of your choice, and continue to condition, condition, condition your hair.

Question 10
How can I get my hair to grow faster?

~ There are several things that contribute to hair growth. I don't believe in a magic pill; instead I believe eating healthier, working out, and proper hair care will promote hair growth. Eating foods such as carrots, dark green vegetables, and salmon are awesome. Carrots promote a healthy scalp, dark green veggies such as spinach and broccoli are excellent sources of vitamins A and C, which our bodies need to produce sebum, the scalp's natural hair conditioner. Also, salmon is packed with omega-3 fatty acids. This high-quality protein is filled with the infamous B-12 and iron which aid our hair in growth. Working out reduces stress, which can lead to hair loss, and proper hair care such as washing, conditioning, and hydrating are a must. Overall, keeping a balance of all the things mentioned above will lead to hair growth.

The following are key: **Wash it!** Don't believe the hype that dirt will help your hair grow. Washing your scalp properly and ridding it of dirt and oil build-up are essential for maximum hair growth. You'll also want to make sure that you clean your hair strands of any product build-up which includes oils, silicones, or gels.

Detangle! This is very important for the sisters who have type 3 to 4 hair. If your hair falls within these hair types, detangling will help the styling and manipulation process less stressful on your hair. ALWAYS detangle your natural hair while it's wet. Styling your hair while it's dry, even with a detangler, may cause breakage. Water is a natural lubricant and it adds moisture to your hair as well.

Even if you have very soft or fine hair, detangling you hair is a good step in your hair maintenance process.

I simply encourage women with coarse hair to make this part of their regimen very consistent because of the thickness and the fragility of the hair.

And lastly: **Deep Condition It!**

Deep conditioning is all about quality time. I normally deep condition my hair when I have the extra thirty minutes or an hour to saturate my hair with my favorite deep conditioner and/or hot oil treatment. After placing the conditioner onto the damp hair, you will place a plastic cap over the hair and sit under a dryer for 15 to 30 minutes. If you're not a fan of the hairdryer, you can easily place the cap onto the damp conditioned hair for 45 minutes and do some of those long forgotten chores around the house. Another method for deep conditioning the hair is using the "hot towel" method. Get your towel as warm as you can handle and wrap it around your already damp and conditioned hair. Heat from the hair dryer and towel helps the conditioner to penetrate into your hair strands, leaving your hair moisturized and manageable.

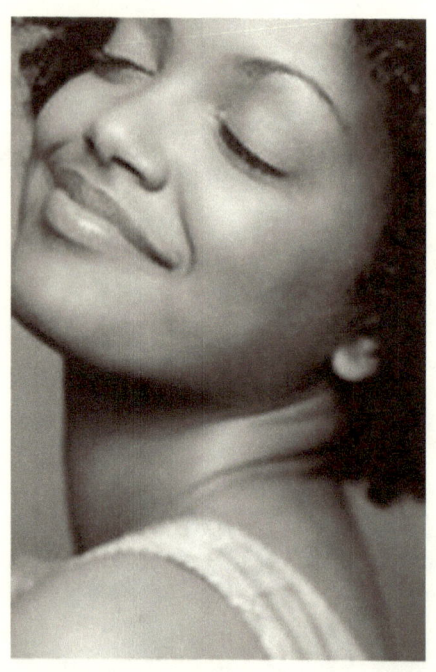

"Beauty is how you feel inside, and it reflects in your eyes. It is not something physical." ~Sophia Loren

CHAPTER 7 ~ NATURALLY YOU FOR LIFE
Know Your Source, And Who You Are

I am so excited for you! Not just because of your decision to go natural, but because of the freedom you will receive on your own journey.

Like all journeys, you will have easy and wide roads as well as narrow and straight roads, but above it all, this journey will be your journey; so take a deep breath and hold on tight. There is something I want you to understand while traveling life journey:

Life is not about your status, it's not about if people like you or dislike you, it's not even about your hair. Life is about love. Loving yourself, loving your family, loving your enemies, and most importantly loving our Creator (God Almighty).

I want you to realize that in order for your crown to shine, you have to shine, and in order for you to shine, you must know who you are and who you belong to. So many women seek refuge in the tangible, but that never tends to be where refuge is found.

People in general have the mentality of, "If I cannot see it, then it is not real". Everything in life has always been about choices, and behind each choice comes action. Think about it, as you said to yourself when you made the decisions to go natural, "Forget this - I'm just going to cut this hair!" As you picked up those scissors or headed to your beautician, you were making a choice.

Your choice led you to act, and your action led to your freedom. Your choice was and is for the betterment of you. Remember, whenever you choose to do something to better yourself there will always be sacrifice. If you are eating healthier, there will be times when you will have to pass on the chocolate cake. If your goal is to lose 10 pounds, you will have to work out an extra 15 minutes.

Nothing worth having or doing comes easy. I am reminded by a sermon I heard from my pastor entitled, "The 3 F's of an Effective Ministry". Well we're going to apply these F's to you and your decision to go natural. The apostle Paul in 2 Timothy 4:7 says, "I have fought the good fight, I have finished the race, I have kept the faith." The first "F" stands for Fought. When you think of this word "fought or fight", you think of a battle between two or more people.

Honestly, there is a battle that we fight every day, and it is in the mind. We struggle with what we know to be right, versus going along to get along. We struggle with making the decision of letting go to live versus holding on while dying. Though we feel it has been so, our fight has never really been with others, but rather it has been with ourselves.

Let us look within and evaluate our reason in wanting natural hair. Is it a fad for you? Are you starting anew? Maybe your goal is to see yourself in a new light and prepare your mind to accept the reflection in the mirror. Whatever your reason, let it come from a place of sincerity and truth, for that will be the best motivator for you as you journey along. I pray it is simply and naturally you.

The second "F" stands for Finished. My pastor gave an analogy of five people being in a race. He stated, "You have never seen someone give up during a race and get a reward". He pretended to run, and as a he slowed down as if he was giving up, he said, "People that continue to run are passing me by and they made it to the finish line - some may have come in third, fourth, or even fifth place, but the goal was to Finish. On your natural hair race, it does not matter if you started your run three years ago or three months ago - keep running and finish your race.

Finishing for you will mean achieving your expectations for your hair. We as women are guilty of comparing our hair to other sisters' hair. We say, 'I went natural at the same time and her hair is longer than mine,' and we become discouraged and give up because we have taken our eyes off of the prize. If your goal is to achieve longer, healthier hair, please believe it can happen.

Stop comparing your hair with others. Believe me, it will become frustrating, and you will give up. You are different; therefore your hair type, hair pattern, and hair growth is different, but the truth still remains, that healthy hair is growing hair. It will grow and probably surpass your expectations. Believe it or not you already have fans. Secret fans I call them.

There are women who wish they were bold enough to take the *leap of faith.* Some women are watching you and admiring you from a distance, maybe even in your circle of friends. So be sure of your decision and be sure of yourself. Finish your race for you, finish your race to be free, and finish your race to free someone else. I pray your race is simply and naturally you.

The third "F" stands for Faith. Now, I know you may be thinking, "What does *faith* have to do with hair?" In the beginning of any journey you cannot see what the end will be. That is why during your process of having natural hair you have to trust and simply believe that your hair will become stronger and healthier.

Having faith in anything is simply believing in something that does not already exist in the natural. I can remember my first attempt. I had just graduated college (and it was not your normal four years). It was more like seven because of my wonderful children and working here and there, but I Finished! So I thought to myself, "If I can complete college with three children, a husband, and a full-time job, surely I can tackle this hair."

I wanted to challenge myself, I wanted something different, and most importantly I did not want anything or anyone to define who I am as a woman.

We should be defined by our integrity. Integrity being who you are when no one is looking. Your hair is there to accentuate your sense of style and your inner self being brought to the surface.

I am not saying women who have permed hair don't know who they are, but what I am saying is, know who you are and expect a great end, no matter how your journey begins.

So have faith my sister, have faith my Queen, and start your journey being simply and naturally you!

Reflections of Chapter 7

1. In order for your crown to shine, _____ have to shine and in order for you to shine, you must know _____ you are and _____ you belong too.

2. Nothing worth _____ or _____ comes easy.

3. True/False: Integrity is who I am when no one is looking.

Write down how your natural hair journey will begin and end.

_____

_____

_____

_____

_____

~APPENDIX A~
The Natural Hair Quiz

1. When I wash my hair it tends to:
   a. draw up
   b. curl up
   c. lay flat

2. When my hair has no oil on it, it feels:
   a. very rough; brittle
   b. dry; yet soft
   c. soft

3. After I apply a moisturizer to my hair it becomes:
   a. soft
   b. very soft
   c. somewhat oily

4. After styling my hair, its shine is:
   a. it doesn't have a shine
   b. somewhat noticeable
   c. very noticeable

5. If I press my hair, it tends to:
   a. lay flat
   b. curl on its own
   c. be bone straight

If you answered mostly a's, you would be considered a 4 which is known as kinky. Kinky hair is very tightly curled, very wiry, very tightly coiled and very, very fragile. It can range from fine/thin to wiry/coarse with lots and lots of strands densely packed together. Type 4 hair is known to shrink up to 75% of the actual hair length especially when wet. Healthy Type 4 hair won't shine, but it will have sheen. With the proper care and technique, type 4 hair is indeed resilient, manageable, durable, growable and easy to control. There are two types, 4A and 4B. 4A has an "S" shaped pattern and 4B has a "Z" shaped pattern.

If you answered mostly b's, you would be considered a 3 which is known as curly. Curly hair has three sub-categories. 3a (big, loose spiral curls), 3b (bouncy ringlets), and 3c (tight corkscrews). Curly hair is the most temperamental hair type. If you apply too much styling product it causes the hair to be weighed down/greasy looking curls; if you apply too little styling products it will be dry and puffy (like a blow out). The key to guaranteeing effortless, frizz-free curls is proper styling product application.

If you answered mostly c's you would be considered a 2 which is known as wavy. Wavy hair also has 3 categories. 2a wavy is fine and thin. It is very easy to handle; easily straightened or curled. 2b is medium textured and has little resistance to styling; also has a tendency to frizz. 2c is thick and coarse, is more resistant to styling, and will frizz easily.

Use lighter products such as mousses or gels that enhance curls, but don't weigh them down. Do not use a brush or comb on your dry curls, and reduce tangles by sleeping on a satin pillowcase.

I did not add a category 1 since my focus is on African American natural hair and I am well aware of those women who may be bi-racial and have a mixture of type 1 and 2 hair. So here is a glimpse of type 1 hair. There are three categories. 1A hair tends to be fine, thin, and very soft. You are likely to have little or no curls- bone straight. 1B hair is medium textured having a lot of body, easy to curl and 1C hair is coarse being resistant to curling and shaping, but also similar to 1A hair in being bone straight.

PRODUCTS FOR EACH HAIR TYPE

I wish someone would have told me about "hair types." It would have saved me time and so..... much money. I hope these products are of great service for your crown and your wallet.

Type 4a/b: (Kinky)

Aubrey Organics Honeysuckle Rose Moisturizing Shampoo
Aubrey Organics Honeysuckle Rose Moisturizing Conditioner
Jane Carter Solution Nourish & Shine
Jane Carter Solution Revitalizing Leave-In Conditioner
Miss Jessie's Curly Pudding 8oz.

Type 3a/b (Curly):

AG Re:coil Curl Activating Shampoo
AG Re:coil Curl Activating Conditioner
Curly Hair Solutions Curl Keeper
Curl Junkie Coffee Coco Curl Creme Lite
Curl Junkie BeautiCurls Daily Hair Conditioner

Type 3c (Tight Curls):

Aubrey Organics White Camellia Ultra-Smoothing Shampoo
Aubrey Organics White Camellia Ultra-Smoothing Conditioner
Aubrey Organics Sea Buckthorn Leave-In Conditioner
Kinky-Curly Knot Today
MYHoneyChild 3-4 Combo Hair Crème

Type 2 (Wavy):

CurlFriends Seduce Pomade
DevaCurl Low-Poo
DevaCurl One Condition
DevaCurl Mist-er Right
DevaCurl Heaven in Hair

Visit **www.secretsofgoingnatural.com/hairproducts** for links to discounts and FREE shipping for these products.

~APPENDIX B~
Products I Love!

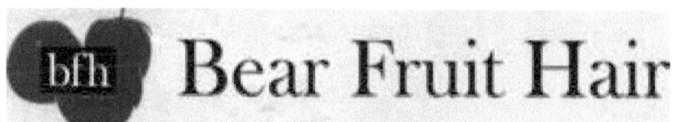

Bear Fruit Products: (www.bearfruithair.com)

Desert Moisturizer & Leave-In Conditioner
Shea Almond Coconut Deep Cream Conditioner
African Export Leave-In Conditioner
360 Scalp Oil

<u>IMPORTANT:</u> Use my personal discount code: **QUEENZ**
anytime you order and get 10% off your entire order.

ORGANIC ROOT Stimulator®
Olive Oil Neutralizing Shampoo
Olive Oil Replenishing Conditioner
Olive Oil Incredibly Rich Moisturizing Hair Lotion

organix.
beauty ○ pure and simple

Organix Nourishing Coconut Milk Shampoo
Organix Nourishing Coconut Milk Conditioner
Nourishing Coconut Milk Anti-Breakage Serum

Visit www.secretsofgoingnatural.com/hairproducts for links
to discounts and **FREE** shipping for these products.

~APPENDIX C~
Interview Links

Visit www.secretsofgoingnatural.com/interviews

To view these and many other videos

Video Interview # 1: **Mrs. Markietta Banks**
3b/c hair type

Video Interview # 2: **Ms. Karin Reeder**
4a hair type

Video Interview # 3: **Dr. Lydia Franklin**
4a/b hair type

Audio Interview # 4: **Carolyn Malachi**
Grammy Nominated, Neo-Soul Singer
4a hair type

~APPENDIX D~
The Truth About Perms

Chemically based products have been around for more than 100 years. Madame C.J.Walker and Garret A. Morgan were the top contributors to the unveiling and overall success of relaxers. Altering the natural state of the hair was thought of as a good thing.

When Madame Walker was confronted with the idea that she was trying to conform black women's hair to that of whites, she stressed that her products were simply an attempt to help black women take proper care of their hair and promote its growth. This statement was her reality and for many women today it still exist, but the truth remain that in fact using a relaxer damages our hair instead of caring for it.

Relaxing our hair causes breakage, scalp irritation, stunted hair growth, and even permanent hair loss. So what exactly does the term "relaxer" mean and what are the overall effects of using these chemicals? A relaxer is a type of lotion or cream which makes hair less curly, and easier to straighten by chemically "relaxing" the natural curls.

The main ingredient in a relaxer is sodium hydroxide. Sodium Hydroxide is a strong alkaline, white compound also known as caustic soda. This white compound permeates the protein structure of the hair and weakens its internal bonds, causing the natural curls to loosen out as the entire fiber swells open. This chemical is also widely used in household cleaning products such as: drain cleaners and oven cleaners.

In applying this cream to your hair you are stripping away its natural oils which are used to maintain moisture. Many women also face alopecia from relaxing the hair. Alopecia means loss of hair from the head sometimes to the extent of baldness.

So now you see the many disadvantages of relaxing your hair.

Make Money With This Book

The Secrets Of Going Natural

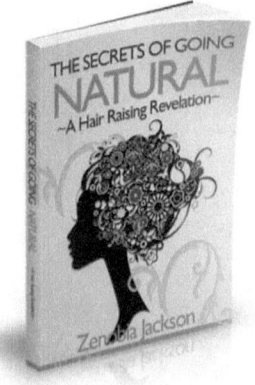

<u>FREE</u> Affiliate Program
Pays 50% Commissions!

Dear Natural Sister,

If you're interested in receiving huge commission payments by simply referring others to this book then all you have to do is sign up for my FREE affiliate program and you can earn some cash while helping another sister who wants to go natural.

Our affiliate program runs through ClickBank (eBook version) and Amazon.com (Kindle Edition or Hard Copy). If you don't have an account already, you'll need to sign up for a free account at each site:

http://clickbank.com
https://affiliate-program.amazon.com

Your Promo Link for ClickBank: (Replace The "CBID" With Your ClickBank ID)

http://CBID.naturallyz.hop.clickbank.net

Here is a great way to make more commissions. Simply **replace the CBID with your ClickBank ID** and promote that link in your emails, articles, blog posts, tweets, .. where ever you want.

Thank you for taking the time to read this page and I hope you have great success promoting Secrets of Going Natural. **Here's To Healthy Natural Hair!**

Sincerely,

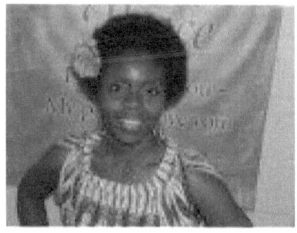

Zenobia Jackson

P.S. - If you have any questions, please email me: NaturallyZee@gmail.com

REFERENCES

Da Costa, Diane. *Textured Tresses*. New York: Fireside Simon & Schuster, 2004.

"Hair Types." Naturallycurly.com. 1998-2011. NaturallyCurly.com, Inc. http://www.naturallycurly.com/hair-types

ABOUT THE AUTHOR

Zenobia Jackson is a happy wife, mother of three, and servant of the Lord. She began her natural journey three years ago and has since learned how to care for and manage her natural hair. Now she is on a personal journey to help as many women as possible take the next steps to realizing their natural beauty.